Evaluation of Instructor and Range Officer Exposure to Emissions from Copper-Based Frangible Ammunition at a Military Firing Range

Mark M. Methner, PhD, CIH
John Gibbins, DVM, MPH
Todd Niemeier, MS, CIH

I0426141

HealthHazard Evaluation Program

Report No. 2012-0091-3187
July 2013

U.S. Department of Health and Human Services
Centers for Disease Control and Prevention
National Institute for Occupational Safety and Health

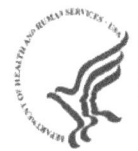
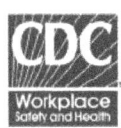
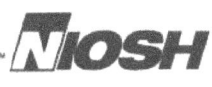

Contents

The cover photo is a close-up image of sorbent tubes, which are used by the HHE Program to measure airborne exposures. This photo is an artistic representation that may not be related to this Health Hazard Evaluation.

Highlights of this Evaluation

The Health Hazard Evaluation Program received a request from a military firing range in North Dakota. The range managers submitted the request because of concern about instructor and range officer exposure to weapons emissions during qualification sessions inside the partially-enclosed firing range. We measured exposure to weapons emissions and assessed health symptoms related to the firing of copper-based ammunition that breaks into pieces on impact (known as frangible ammunition).

What We Did

- We sampled the air for contaminants in weapons emissions during firing events that occurred in February 2012–March 2012.

- We interviewed instructors and range officers and documented their health complaints and concerns.

- We measured airflow inside the firing range.

- We observed the instructors' and range officer's work practices.

- We reviewed medical records, health questionnaires, and reports about instructor and student symptoms.

- We talked with engineering, public health, and flight surgeon staff about prior evaluations of the firing range.

What We Found

- Air contaminant concentrations did not exceed occupational exposure limits.

- The ventilation system was not designed to remove air contaminants.

> We assessed instructor and range officer exposure to emissions from weapons during firing events at a military firing range. No exposures exceeded occupational exposure limits, yet instructors and range officers continued to report health symptoms. The ventilation system was not designed to remove air contaminants. We recommended modifying the system to improve removal of air contaminants or constructing an enclosed range with a suitable ventilation system to control air contaminants.

- Firing weapons when the propane-fired heater was on produced higher carbon monoxide levels than the heater itself produced.

- Levels of very small particles inside the range increased during firing events.

- Some instructors did not wear protective eyewear, or they wore eyewear without side shields.

- Instructors reported symptoms such as headache, metallic taste, sore throat, and respiratory symptoms they felt were associated with the firing of frangible ammunition.

- The symptoms instructors told us about were similar to those reported by instructors in previous surveys at this facility. They are consistent with the types of exposures that we measured.

What We Found (continued)

- Some shooters did not wear hearing protection correctly.
- Some instructors consumed drinks inside the range.
- Some instructors did not wash their hands before eating or smoking after firing events.

What the Employer Can Do

- Modify the ventilation system so that air contaminants are exhausted out of the range.
- Inspect and adjust the propane-fired heater to reduce the amount of carbon monoxide it produces.
- Remind staff periodically on the proper use and type of hearing protection.
- Require all eyewear worn inside the range to be fitted with side shields.
- Rotate range duties, if possible, to minimize time spent inside the range during firing events.

What Employees Can Do

- Report symptoms and health concerns to your supervisor.
- If you get medical care, tell your healthcare provider and the public health office that you work at the firing range.
- Do not drink or eat inside the range.
- If you wear protective eyewear during firing events, make sure side shields are attached.
- Wash hands before eating or smoking.
- Participate in programs to help you stop smoking.

Mention of any company or product does not constitute endorsement by NIOSH. In addition, citations to websites external to NIOSH do not constitute NIOSH endorsement of the sponsoring organizations or their programs or products. Furthermore, NIOSH is not responsible for the content of these websites. All web addresses referenced in this document were accessible as of the publication date of this report.

Abbreviations

μm	Micrometer
$\mu g/m^3$	Micrograms per cubic meter
ACGIH®	American Conference of Governmental Industrial Hygienists
BEI	Biological exposure index
CFR	Code of Federal Regulations
CO	Carbon monoxide
IOM	Institute of Medicine
Lpm	Liters per minute
mg/m^3	Milligrams per cubic meter
mm	Millimeter
NA	Not applicable
ND	Not detected
NIOSH	National Institute for Occupational Safety and Health
nm	Nanometer
OEL	Occupational exposure limit
OSHA	Occupational Safety and Health Administration
PEL	Permissible exposure limit
PM	Particulate mass
ppm	Parts per million
REL	Recommended exposure limit
TLV®	Threshold limit value
TWA	Time-weighted average

Introduction

The Health Hazard Evaluation Program received a request from the managers of a military firing range in North Dakota. The request concerned potential occupational exposure of training instructors and range officers to copper particulate and gases/aerosols/irritants during qualification sessions involving the firing of frangible copper ammunition from small arms (M4 rifle using 5.56 millimeter [mm] rounds and M9 handgun using 9 millimeter rounds). We evaluated the facility in February–March 2012. We observed instructor and range officer work practices, evaluated the firing range heating and ventilation system, and measured airborne levels of copper particulate, irritant gases, carbon monoxide (CO), and particle number and mass concentrations inside the range. In August 2012, an interim report outlining our preliminary findings and recommendations was sent to the requestor, the supervisor of the firing range, and the facility health and safety department.

Background

Ammunition

Historically, lead has been used in the manufacture of bullets. However, because of environmental and human health concerns, the use of lead ammunition has declined. Over the last decade, this range opted to use lead-free frangible ammunition for small arms training with M4 and M9 weapons. The frangible ammunition was considered nontoxic because lead was no longer present in the bullet or the primer. Also, the frangible bullet presents less ricochet hazard because it is designed to fragment upon impact. The frangible bullets evaluated during this assessment were made of compacted metal powder (95% copper; 5% zinc).

Training Sessions

Shooters were required to complete two phases of qualification. Phase 1 qualification consisted of each shooter discharging six magazines, each containing four rounds, with the M4 rifle at a target 25 meters downrange until it was deemed "zeroed in" by the firing line instructor. Once the weapon was zeroed, new targets were installed by the instructors, and each shooter then discharged the following: 1 magazine with 5 rounds, 1 magazine with 10 rounds (5 live/5 blank), and 20 magazines with 3 rounds. Each of the firing events occurred from different shooting positions (e.g., prone, standing, kneeling).

Phase 2 qualification, typically done the following day, involved each shooter firing the zeroed weapon from different shooting positions at targets ranging from 3 to approximately 25 meters downrange. Each shooter discharged the following: 1 magazine with 12 rounds, 2 magazines with 5 rounds, 3 magazines with 8 rounds, 2 magazines with 9 rounds, 6 magazines with 4 rounds, 1 magazine with 6 rounds, and 4 magazines with 2 rounds. At the conclusion of Phase 2, each shooter's target was graded by a firing line instructor who determined whether the shooter was successful in the qualification attempt.

In addition to the Phase 1 and 2 qualification sessions, two other types of weapons training occurred during our evaluation. One involved firing 30 rounds with the M4 and 30 rounds with the M9. Another training session involved firing 100 rounds using just the M9.

Firing Range

The range was a wooden structure on a concrete slab. It had 28 shooting lanes, each with split doors (upper and lower segments) that allowed shooters to fire at targets located under an outdoor ballistic canopy. A ventilation system heated the range during cold weather. A main air supply duct ran the length of the range and a direct fire propane burner was in-line midway along the main duct. Outdoor air was drawn into the heater via a roof-mounted intake. As air moved into the system, it was heated by the propane burner and discharged along the length of the supply duct via eight ducts that extended perpendicularly from the main duct to the back wall of the range. Each supply duct pointed down and discharged air through a louvered rectangular supply register (Figure 1).

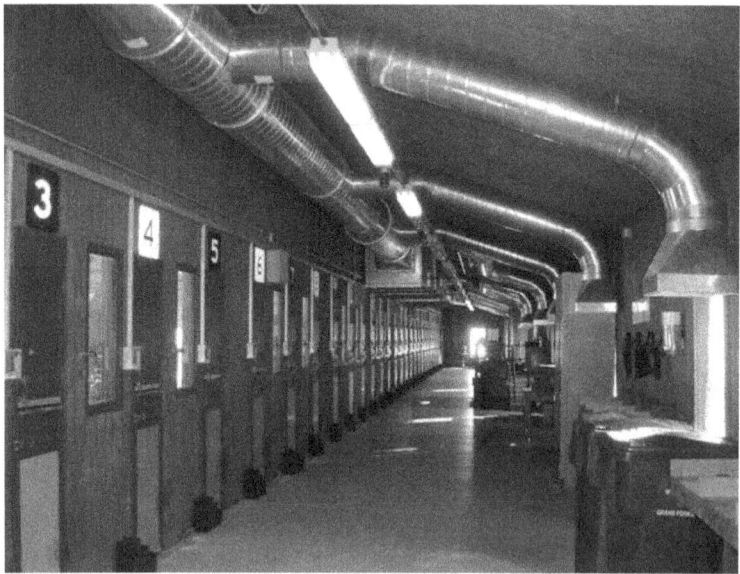

Figure 1. Firing range layout and heating/ventalation system at the time of the evaluation.

We reviewed the results from a January 2009 health survey of nine range instructors and students. All nine instructors reported runny nose, chest tightness, watery eyes, cough, and headache usually during or immediately after an exposure firing event. Among the students, 7 of 47 (15%) reported similar symptoms. These results, along with prior complaints and concerns about exposures at the range, prompted the decision to modify the ventilation system.

Methods

Objectives

1. Measure instructor and range officer exposures to air contaminants generated by firing copper frangible ammunition.

2. Characterize the particle number, size, shape, and chemical composition of the aerosol.

3. Evaluate the ventilation system to determine effectiveness in removing air contaminants.

4. Determine whether exposure to air contaminants is linked to health symptoms reported by instructors and range officers.

Air Sampling

Task-based personal and area air samples for elemental analysis were collected during office/classroom work and qualification sessions using a 37-mm open-faced cassette containing a 0.8-micrometer (µm) mixed cellulose ester filter. The filter cassette was attached to a personal sampling pump operating at 2 liters per minute (Lpm). Personal air sampling devices were attached to the lapel of a firing line instructor, range officer, classroom instructor, and shooter. Area air samples were collected 3 feet above the floor on a shelf midway between firing lanes (1-15), approximately 8 feet behind the firing line. All samples were analyzed by the National Institute for Occupational Safety and Health (NIOSH) Method 7303 [NIOSH 2013].

Additional air samples were collected on firing line instructors, range officers, classroom instructors, and some shooters during qualification sessions using the Institute of Medicine (IOM) inhalable particle sampler. These samplers were outfitted with a MultiDust™ polyurethane foam prefilter followed by a 25-mm mixed cellulose ester filter [SKC Inc. 2013]. The foam prefilter allowed us to measure inhalable and respirable fractions [Mohlmann et al. 2002; SKC Inc. 2013]. The sample collected on the foam was analyzed separately and added to the result obtained for the mixed cellulose ester filter to determine the inhalable fraction of the aerosol [SKC Inc. 2013]. We did not collect air samples specifically for copper fume. However, it is reasonable to compare the respirable copper particulate concentration to the copper fume occupational exposure limits (OELs) because the respirable particulate and fume are similar in size. Area air samples were also collected using the IOM sampler with the polyurethane prefilter. We used a flow rate of 2 Lpm, and each IOM sample was analyzed for elements using NIOSH Method 7303 [NIOSH 2013].

To examine the morphology, size, and chemical composition of particulate emitted during weapon firing, personal and area air samples were collected using 37-mm, 0.8-µm pore size mixed cellulose ester filters and analyzed via transmission electron microscopy using a modification of NIOSH Method 7402 (direct air method) [NIOSH 2013]. The modification consisted of using a portion of each filter and affixing it to a glass slide using a clearing solution (35% dimethyl formamide, 15% glacial acetic acid, and 50% deionized water). Once cleared, each filter was carbon coated and placed onto three 200 mesh nickel grids without plasma ashing. Each grid was viewed under various magnifications (15,000X or higher) using a FEI/Philips CM-12 microscope equipped with an integrated x-ray fluorescence digital imaging system (FEI/Philips Electron Optics). The microscopist examined at least 40 grid openings or 100 particles, whichever came first, and captured a digital image of the particulate. Energy dispersive spectrometry was used to identify the chemical composition of the particles observed.

Airborne particle number concentration and particle mass concentration were measured with two different instruments. Particle number concentration across the size range of 20 nanometers (nm) to 1,000 nm was measured in the area near the firing line using a TSI P-Trak® Model 8525 real-time, datalogging device. The particle mass air concentration was measured using the TSI Dust Trak® DRX Model 8533 aerosol photometer, which responds to particulate in the range of 0.001 milligrams per cubic meter of air (mg/m^3) to 150 mg/m^3.

This instrument simultaneously measures size-segregated particulate mass (PM) fractions corresponding to 1 μm (PM1), 2.5 μm (PM2.5), respirable (4 μm), 10 μm (PM10) and 100 μm (total PM) size fractions.

Area air concentrations of CO, nitric oxide, and nitrogen dioxide were measured using a BW Technologies Gas Alert Extreme® instrument.

Thermal desorption tubes were used to collect area air samples to identify volatile organic compounds using NIOSH Method 2549 [NIOSH 2013]. Based on these results we used charcoal tubes to quantify the air concentration of volatile organic compounds in accordance with NIOSH Method 1300 [NIOSH 2013]. Task-based area air samples using silica gel tubes were collected at a flow rate of 200 cubic centimeters per minute and analyzed for inorganic acids (hydrobromic, hydrochloric, hydrofluoric, nitric, phosphoric, and sulfuric) using NIOSH Method 7903 [NIOSH 2013]. Dräger® colorimetric detector tube samples were collected near the instructors midway through two firing events to estimate air concentrations of phosgene, ammonia, hydrochloric acid, and hydrogen cyanide.

Ventilation assessment

We characterized the airflow patterns created by the ventilation system and measured the centerline air velocity at each firing lane doorway using a TSI Velocicalc® Plus model 8386A anemometer. Triplicate measurements were collected at each shooting lane door opening at two heights (approximately 3 feet and 5 feet). To visualize airflow patterns created by the ventilation system, we used a Rosco Laboratories Inc. fog-generating machine.

Interviews

We held voluntary, confidential interviews with all 12 enlisted personnel assigned to the range. This included instructors, range officers, armory personnel, and instructor trainees. On February 28, 2012, we met with the flight surgeon, engineering officer in charge and staff, and the public health officer in charge and staff to discuss their past involvement with the firing range and review records. We reviewed records, including five medical records from personnel who reported seeking medical care for their symptoms and three occupational illness/injury reports filed in January 2009/2010 for range instructors. We also reviewed copies and summaries of health symptom surveys that had been administered by the public health officer to range students and instructors.

Results

Air sampling

During our evaluation 63 shooters completed the qualification course, discharging 6,904 frangible bullet rounds. Eight individuals served as firing line instructors, range officers, or classroom instructors during 5 days of sampling. Many of the instructors and range officers rotated roles during qualification sessions. For example, an instructor working the firing line during the morning session served as the range officer during the afternoon session.

We collected 127 task-based and shorter-term air samples during seven weapon qualification sessions and longer-term air samples during office/classroom activities. For firing line instruction and range officer work, task-based sampling times ranged from 26 to 142 minutes. Sampling times ranged from 210 to 386 minutes for office/classroom work. OELs for copper are presented in Table 1.

Table 1. OELs for copper in air samples ($\mu g/m^3$)

	Dusts/Mists	Copper (Inhalable)	Copper (Fume)
NIOSH REL	1,000	NA	100
OSHA PEL	1,000	NA	100
ACGIH TLV	1,000	NA	200
MAC (Netherlands)	NA	100	NA
MAK (Germany-DFG)	NA	100	NA
MAK (Germany-DFG)	NA	200*	NA

$\mu g/m^3$ = micrograms per cubic meter, ACGIH = American Conference of Governmental Industrial Hygienists, NA = not applicable, OSHA = Occupational Safety and Health Administration, REL = recommended exposure limit (up to 10 hours), PEL= permissible exposure limit (eight hour time-weighted average), TLV = threshold limit value (eight hour time-weighted average), MAC (Netherlands) = maximum allowable concentration for inhalable copper particulate, MAK (Germany-DFG) = maximum eight hour time-weighted average.

*MAK (Germany-DFG) for short-term 15 minute average.

None of the personal air samples collected on instructors, range officers or shooters exceeded any applicable occupational exposure limit for copper (Table 2). Total copper concentrations for instructors ranged from not detected (ND) to 26 $\mu g/m^3$ while concentrations for range officers were much lower (range = ND to 4.5 $\mu g/m^3$). The three shooters had total copper concentrations that ranged from 9–24 $\mu g/m^3$. Short-term air sample results from three shooters measured higher total copper concentrations when compared to most instructors and all range officers (range = 9 to 24 $\mu g/m^3$) (Appendix A, Table A2). One short-term exposure limit sample collected on a shooter resulted in a copper concentration of 18 $\mu g/m^3$. The eight area air samples had copper concentrations ranging from ND to 19 $\mu g/m^3$ (Appendix A, Table A1). Copper was not detected (< 0.14 $\mu g/m^3$) on air samples collected on instructors or range officers while they were engaged in office/classroom work.

Table 2. Range of task-based copper concentrations (µg/m³) during qualification sessions

Job	Weapon	37-mm cassette total copper	37-mm cassette total copper short-term*	IOM inhalable copper	IOM respirable copper
Instructor N = 14	M4	1.6–26	3.5–16	1.5–19	ND (< 1.5)–15
	M4+M9	ND (< 2.0)	[2.8]	ND (< 2.0)	ND (< 2.0)
	M9	ND (< 1.0)	ND (< 1.7)	ND (< 1.5)	ND (< 1.5)
Range officer N = 7	M4	ND (< 1.0)–4.5	NS	1.0–4.0	1.0–3.8
	M4+M9	ND (< 2.0)	NS	ND (< 2.0)	ND (< 2.0)
	M9	ND (< 1.0)	NS	[3.1]	[2.2]
Shooter N = 3	M4	9–24*	18**	NS	NS

NS = not sampled

*Short-term samples ranged from 7–30 minutes.

**One short-term exposure limit sample collected

Note: Values in parentheses indicate the minimum detectable concentration (MDC) for those samples; values in brackets are between the MDC and the minimum quantifiable concentration (MQC); more uncertainty is associated with these samples.

None of the inhalable or respirable fractions collected with the IOM samplers exceeded their applicable OELs. Range officers generally had lower inhalable copper concentrations than instructors.

All of the personal and area air samples submitted for transmission electron microscopy analysis showed the presence of singular, spherical elemental copper and copper particulate (e.g., copper sulfide) ranging from 50–250 nm in diameter (Appendix B, Figure B1). Zinc and iron particulate in the same size range were found but copper was more prevalent.

As shown in Appendix B, Figure B2, the particle number concentration in the 20–1,000 nm size range measured with the P-Trak instrument rapidly increased during firing events. The same pattern was observed when measuring the area particle mass air concentration using the Dust Trak instrument (Appendix B, Figure B3).

The CO concentration averaged 8 parts per million (ppm) (range: 4–23 ppm) during firing events with the heat on and the shooting lane doors open (Appendix B, Figures B4 and B5). With the heat on and the shooting doors closed (no firing), the CO concentration averaged 13 ppm. Once the shooting doors were opened, the CO concentration decreased to an average of 6 ppm but when firing began, the CO concentration increased quickly, peaking at 23 ppm (Appendix B, Figures B4 and B5). These concentrations are below the OSHA time-weighted average (TWA) permissible exposure limit of 50 ppm and NIOSH ceiling limit of 200 ppm. Nitric oxide concentrations averaged 0.3 ppm and nitrogen dioxide concentrations averaged 0.2 ppm; both were well below their applicable OELs.

No volatile organic compounds related to the firing of weapons were detected on the thermal desorption tube air samples. Concentrations of hydrobromic, hydrochloric, hydrofluoric, nitric, phosphoric, and sulfuric acids were below their respective OELs (Appendix A, Table A3). Phosgene, ammonia, hydrochloric acid, and hydrogen cyanide were not detected on colorimetric detector tubes during two firing events.

Ventilation assessment

Air velocities at the door opening of each of the shooting lanes 1–15 (those in use during firing events) ranged from 50 feet per minute to approximately 200 feet per minute. Air velocities in shooting lanes 16–28 (not used during the assessment) were higher, and more variable (range = 98 to 307 feet per minute). These measurements are higher than the NIOSH recommended range of 50 to 75 feet per minute for indoor firing ranges [NIOSH 2009]. With the ventilation system operating and using the fog-generating machine, airflow appeared to be turbulent and circular. The supply duct directed air downward towards the floor. The air then moved along the floor toward the shooting lane door opening, moved up the wall toward the ceiling, and then moved back toward the rear wall. Very little air was observed exiting the shooting lane door openings. We also observed, on occasion, fog exiting one doorway and re-entering an adjacent doorway.

Observations

We saw some range officers and instructors consuming beverages in the range. Some range officers and instructors did not wash their hands after leaving the range. We also saw some instructors and students wearing eyewear without protective side shields and some students wearing foam insert ear plugs incorrectly.

Interviews

The 12 personnel we interviewed had been assigned to this range for an average of 20 months (range: 2 weeks to 54 months). All reported one or more health symptoms (Table 3). Five instructors reported working for brief periods (typically 2–4 months on average) at other firing ranges. One of the five reported acute upper respiratory symptoms while at another firing range. Nearly all (11 of 12) reported that symptoms occurred within 1–2 hours after firing commenced. Most personnel said that symptoms typically improved within hours after the firing ended. One employee said that his symptoms lasted until the next day and recurred if he worked on the firing line that day.

When asked what conditions contributed to their symptoms, 9 of 12 reported symptoms were more likely to occur with a larger class size. Most had symptoms when at least 6–8 students were in the class. Other contributing factors mentioned were night-fire classes, northerly wind direction that resulted in weapon emissions being directed back into the range, and firing the M4 weapon. Five of 12 reported seeking medical care primarily for headache and respiratory symptoms either at the facility's medical clinic or at an urgent care facility. Two instructors reported instances where students had previously complained about nausea during class.

Table 3. Self-reported health symptoms by range personnel, February 27–28, 2012

Health symptom	Number of personnel reporting symptoms	Percent (%)
Headache	11/12	92
"Bad" metallic taste	5/12	42
Sore throat	4/12	33
Shortness of breath	3/12	25
Nasal/sinus irritation	3/12	25
Nausea	1/12	8

Note: Some personnel reported more than one symptom.

We learned that on October 6, 2010, 15 students using the firing range were given a health symptom survey. We reviewed these surveys and summarized the results. When asked if they developed any symptoms during or within 30 minutes of ending training, 5 of 15 reported symptoms, 8 of 15 reported no symptoms, and 2 of 15 did not respond. Among those reporting symptoms, 4 of 5 reported itchy, watery eyes, and 2 of 5 reported sore/scratchy throat. Headache and "bad" metallic taste, the symptoms most commonly reported during our instructor interviews, were not listed choices on the student survey. All personnel who reported symptoms reported that their symptoms resolved in less than a day after training. Additionally, we analyzed the results of surveys administered to five range personnel by the public health office on September 23–24, 2010. All five personnel reported having symptoms either during or within 30 minutes of the end of training. Reported symptoms were similar to the results of our February 2012 interviews and included headache, cough, sore throat, and other respiratory symptoms. Symptoms were reported to occur most of the time during training by four of five instructors, and all instructors reported symptoms resolved within hours to one day after the class.

We discussed the range medical surveillance program and confirmed that annual audiograms were the only medical test administered to range personnel, on the basis of prior risk assessment and industrial hygiene sampling. We reviewed three occupational illness/injury reports that were completed by the flight surgeon in January 2009 and 2010. These three range personnel sought medical care for headache, nausea, vomiting, and cough that occurred during weapons firing at the range. A determination of work-related illness was made on the basis of temporal association of symptoms to weapons firing. No specific diagnosis or additional medical follow-up was documented on these forms.

We reviewed medical records for five range instructors who reported seeking medical care for symptoms they experienced during weapons firing at the range. These five instructors were seen by three different healthcare providers, making it difficult to associate symptoms with a specific job or shop. Chronic headaches (occurring periodically for weeks to months when working on the range) were reported by four personnel. All four personnel reported headaches were more common with larger class sizes and were associated with the use of frangible ammunition. Individuals used a variety of over the counter or prescription medication for their headaches. Shortness of breath/wheeze was reported by three instructors.

Two instructors had further medical follow-up with chest x-rays, complete blood count, and metabolic profile, all of which were within normal limits. One instructor had spirometry (lung function) results that were within normal limits, and one was referred for pulmonary follow-up; test results were not available. One instructor was seen for seasonal allergies. All instructors returned to work without restriction of duties.

Discussion

During our assessment of the range, a large volume of monitoring data was collected using direct-reading instruments. Regardless of the weapon fired and the session, day, or amount of ammunition discharged, each instrument showed an increase in airborne contaminants when weapons were fired. These results suggest that the existing ventilation system in the firing range was not effective in controlling emissions from weapons during firing events, resulting in unnecessary exposures for employees working inside the range. Although these contaminants do not exceed any OELs, instructors and range officers consistently reported health symptoms that they believed were related to their exposure during qualification sessions. The results of our air sampling and interviews are consistent with past surveys at this and other similar locations [AFIOH 2008]. Furthermore, the material safety data sheet for the frangible ammunition acknowledges the potential for respiratory irritation. The concentrations of CO and the duration of exposure measured are below the levels typically associated with headache and nausea. Although no contaminants exceeded their OELs, a combination of these exposures could have contributed to reported health symptoms as previously reported in other settings [AFIOH 2008].

The ventilation system at the range was intended for heating, not air contaminant control. We observed that because the range is partially open to the outdoors, wind direction and wind speed created turbulent air movement in the range. This resulted in weapons emissions, on occasion, being directed back into the range. Data from the meteorological office indicated that the prevailing wind direction during our evaluation was mostly from the north (towards the shooters) at speeds ranging from 14 to 29 miles per hour. With substantial wind speed from the north (toward the shooting lane doors), the ventilation system may not be able to remove air contaminants. To account for this situation, an alternative exhaust ventilation system may be needed until a fully enclosed range is constructed. Additionally, the ventilation system needs to be designed to address the CO generated by the propane gas furnace and weapon firing.

One of the objectives of this assessment was to characterize the aerosol generated during firing events. On the basis of the air sampling data and microscopic examination, the aerosol produced during firing events consists primarily of nano- and fume-sized copper particulate. Because this small copper particulate contains little mass but a high surface area it may be more reactive than larger copper particles. The toxicity of nano-sized copper has been studied in cell cultures and in animals. These studies concluded that, because of the small size and increased surface area of the nano-sized particles, inhalation exposure could result in cellular uptake, formation of reactive oxidative species and subsequent inflammation and irritation

[Pettibone et al. 2008; Wang et al. 2012]. This may explain why health symptoms were reported, yet no mass-based OEL was exceeded.

In general, range officers were exposed to less copper than instructors and shooters. This may be because the range officer is located farther away from the firing activity when compared to the instructors and shooters. Also, copper concentrations were generally higher when more rounds were fired. When comparing weapon type and measured concentrations of copper, it appears that the M9 handgun produced less airborne copper particulate than the M4 rifle. This may be due to a smaller amount of copper in the 9 mm bullet and also the shorter barrel length resulting in less opportunity to mechanically abrade or heat the copper bullet and produce particulate as it travels through the barrel.

It should be noted that this evaluation may not be indicative of a worst-case scenario because the range was not fully occupied. Also, variability in airflow out of the range due to changing wind patterns makes drawing definitive conclusions difficult. Furthermore, our evaluation was conducted over a short period of time and different results may be found under different environmental conditions (e.g., wind speed and direction).

Conclusions

Despite measuring exposures that were below OELs, it is possible that reported symptoms are related to emissions generated during weapons firing. An exposure to very small copper particulate (nano-size to fume size), along with other respiratory irritants (acid gases and CO), could result in the health symptoms reported by the instructors and range officers.

During our site visit, range personnel mentioned that construction of an indoor range is scheduled for completion in approximately 3–4 years. Such a facility, if appropriately constructed and ventilated, should further reduce the exposures measured in this evaluation [USN 2002, NIOSH 2009]. However, until a new range is constructed, modifications to the ventilation system are recommended.

Recommendations

On the basis of our findings, we recommend the actions listed. We encourage the facility to create a firing range staff-management working group to discuss our recommendations and develop an action plan. This committee should work closely with the occupational health and safety group. The working group can set priorities and assess the feasibility of our recommendations.

Our recommendations are based on an approach known as the hierarchy of controls (Appendix C). This approach groups actions by their likely effectiveness in reducing or removing hazards. In most cases, the preferred approach is to eliminate hazardous materials or processes and install engineering controls to reduce exposure or shield employees. Until such controls are in place, or if they are not effective or feasible, administrative measures and personal protective equipment may be needed.

Elimination and Substitution

Eliminating or substituting hazardous processes or materials reduces hazards and protects employees more effectively than other approaches. Prevention through design, considering elimination or substitution when designing or developing a project, reduces the need for additional controls in the future. The plans for a new enclosed range would allow for a prevention-through-design approach. However, until such a facility is operational, the following should be considered:

Engineering Controls

Engineering controls reduce employees' exposures by removing the hazard from the process or by placing a barrier between the hazard and the employee. Engineering controls protect employees effectively without placing primary responsibility of implementation on the employee.

1. Consult with a ventilation engineer to determine changes to the ventilation system to ensure that air contaminants are directed out the shooting lane door openings. During warmer months, use the existing air handler in "fan only" mode to provide adequate airflow out of each door opening. If such a modification is not feasible, consider designing and installing an exhaust system capable of removing air contaminants and directing them outdoors.

2. If a modified ventilation system is installed, carry out follow-up exposure assessments with medical interviews and health record reviews to ensure a reduction in exposure and associated health effects.

3. Inspect the liquid propane gas furnace and adjust the burner air/gas mixture so that CO concentrations are as low as reasonably achievable. Install a CO monitor that will provide an audible alarm above a threshold concentration.

Administrative Controls

The term administrative control refers to employer-dictated work practices and policies to reduce or prevent hazardous exposures. Their effectiveness depends on employer commitment and employee acceptance. Regular monitoring and reinforcement are necessary to ensure that policies and procedures are followed consistently.

1. Increase the rotation of instructors and range officers between classroom/office activities and firing line activities. This will reduce their time inside the range during firing.

2. Instruct personnel not to eat or drink while inside the range.

3. Instruct personnel to wash their hands with soap and water immediately after leaving the range area.

4. Ask range personnel to notify the public health office when medical attention is sought from military or civilian personnel because of symptoms they feel may be related to exposures, so appropriate investigation, trend analysis, and follow-up can occur.

5. Encourage range personnel to inform healthcare providers that they work at the range when seeking care for symptoms that may be related to occupational exposure. Healthcare providers should also report these encounters to the public health office for further evaluation in accordance with facility policy.

6. Require managers to participate in health and safety meetings when the range is periodically evaluated. Health and safety team members should be involved in any committees or working groups.

Personal Protective Equipment

Personal protective equipment is the least effective means for controlling hazardous exposures. Proper use of personal protective equipment requires a comprehensive program and a high level of employee involvement and commitment. The right personal protective equipment must be chosen for each hazard. Supporting programs such as training, change-out schedules, and medical assessment may be needed. Personal protective equipment should not be the sole method for controlling hazardous exposures. Rather, personal protective equipment should be used until effective engineering and administrative controls are in place.

1. Provide all range officers, instructors, and students with safety glasses with side shields before they are allowed into the range. Provide attachable side shields for individuals who wear prescription glasses.

2. Instruct students on how to correctly insert foam earplugs. Information on proper technique for inserting foam earplugs can be found on the NIOSH website at http://www.cdc.gov/niosh/mining/content/earplug.html.

3. Use dual hearing protection (earplugs and earmuffs) when firing weapons, provided using these devices do not interfere with the ability to hear instructor and range officer commands [NIOSH 2009].

Appendix A: Tables

Table A1. Total, inhalable, and respirable copper particulate during qualification sessions in 2012

Date	Weapon	Phase and time	No. of shooters/ Rounds fired	Sample time (min)	Sample type	Concentration (µg/m³)		
						Total	Inhalable	Respirable
2-27	M4	1 (pm)	9/846	142	Instr	4.2	4.4	3.5
				142	Instr	18	19	15
				145	RO	4.5	4.0	3.3
				140	Area	9.3	9.5	7.9
2-28	M4	2 (am)	9/918	85	Instr	4.8	5.4	4.4
				81	Instr	[1.9]*	[2.4]	[1.9]
				85	RO	[1.4]	[2.1]	[1.7]
				90	Area	5.6	4.3	3.7
2-28	M4/M9	NA (pm)	7/420	27	Instr	ND (< 2.0)†	NS	NS
				26	Instr	ND (< 2.0)	ND (< 2.0)	ND (< 2.0)
				28	RO	ND (< 2.0)	ND (< 2.0)	ND (< 2.0)
				35	Area	ND (< 2.0)	ND (< 2.0)	ND (< 2.0)
2-29	M9	NA (pm)	8/800	43	Instr	ND (< 1.0)	ND (< 1.5)	ND (< 1.5)
				40	Instr	ND (< 1.0)	ND (< 1.5)	ND (< 1.5)
				45	RO	ND (< 1.0)	[3.1]	[2.2]
				48	Area	ND (< 1.0)	ND (< 1.5)	ND (< 1.5)
3-1	M4	1 + 2 (am)	10/1960	131	Instr	26	15	12
				138	Instr	4.0	[1.8]	[1.5]
				129	RO	3.2	4.5	3.8
				127	Area	19	18	13
3-1	M4	1 (pm)	10/940	131	Instr	8.4	10	7.6
				125	Instr	2.6	2.3	1.7
				131	RO	[1.2]	[0.9]	[0.9]
				132	Area	7.2	ND (< 0.5)	ND (< 0.5)
3-2	M4	2 (am)	10/1020	71	Instr	3.5	[1.5]	[1.2]
				70	Instr	[1.6]	[2.0]	[1.6]
				74	RO	ND (< 1.0)	[1.4]	[1.0]
				69	Area	5.0	[2.0]	[1.9]

Instr = Instructor breathing zone air sample

min = Minutes

RO = Range officer breathing zone air sample

*Results shown in brackets indicate the value is between the MDC and the MQC; more uncertainty is associated with these sample results. Because of different sampling times the MDC for the total particulate samples ranged from 0.13–1.9 µg/m³ and 0.19–1.9 µg/m³ for the IOM samples, and the MQC for the total particulate samples ranged from 1.5–2.3 µg/m³ and 2.5–8 µg/m³ for the IOM samples.

†Values shown in parenthesis indicate the MDC for that sample.

Note: Other metals present on samples but in amounts not quantifiable include barium, zirconium, tellurium, manganese, iron, antimony, chromium, tin, vanadium, potassium, titanium, strontium, aluminum, calcium.

Table A2. Total copper particulate short-term samples in the breathing zone of instructors and shooters during weapon qualification sessions

Date	Weapon	Phase and time	No. of shooters/ Rounds fired	Sampling time (min)	Sample type	Concentration ($\mu g/m^3$)
2-28	M4	2 (am)	9/918	15	Instr	3.5*
				7	Instr	3.9*
2-28	M4+M9	NA (pm)	7/420	15	Instr	[2.8]*†
2-29	M9	NA (pm)	8/800	15	Instr	ND (< 1.7)*
3-1	M4	1+2 (am)	10/1960	16	Instr	16*
				15	Shooter	18*
				27	Shooter	24‡
				28	Shooter	8.6‡
3-1	M4	1 (pm)	10/940	15	Instr	16*
				15	Instr	11*
3-2	M4	2 (am)	10/1020	30	Instr	3.5‡
				25	Instr	4.7‡

*Short-term exposure limit sample

†MDC for this sample was 6.3 $\mu g/m^3$.

‡Short duration sample

Note: Task-based samples resulted in different MDCs and MQCs. Values in parentheses indicate the MDC for those samples; values in brackets are between the MDC and the MQC; more uncertainty is associated with these samples.

Note: Short-term exposure limit samples collected at a flow rate of 4 Lpm.

Note: Other metals present on samples but in amounts not quantifiable include; barium, zirconium, tellurium, manganese, iron, antimony, chromium, tin, vanadium, potassium, titanium, strontium, aluminum, calcium.

Table A3. Acid gases collected on area samples during weapon qualification sessions

Date	Weapon	Phase And Time	No. of shooters/ Rounds fired	Sampling time (min)	Concentration ($\mu g/m^3$)	Comments
2-27	M4	1 (pm)	9/846	141	[170]	Nitric acid MQC = 350
2-28	M4	2 (am)	9/918	90	630	Nitric acid
				90	[180]	Phosphoric acid MQC = 560
				90	[67]	Sulfuric acid MQC = 560
2-28	M4+M9	NA (pm)	7/420	34	190	HCl
2-29	M9	NA (pm)	8/800	44	ND (< 200)	No acids detected
3-1	M4	1+2 (am)	10/1960	128	[130]	Nitric acid MQC = 390
3-1	M4	1 (pm)	10/940	133	[140]	Nitric acid MQC = 380
3-2	M4	2 (pm)	10/1020	71	[170]	Nitric acid MQC = 700

HCl = Hydrochloric acid

Note: Task-based samples resulted in different MDCs and MQCs. Values in parentheses indicate the MDC for those samples; values in brackets are between the MDC and the MQC; more uncertainty is associated with these samples.

Appendix B: Figures

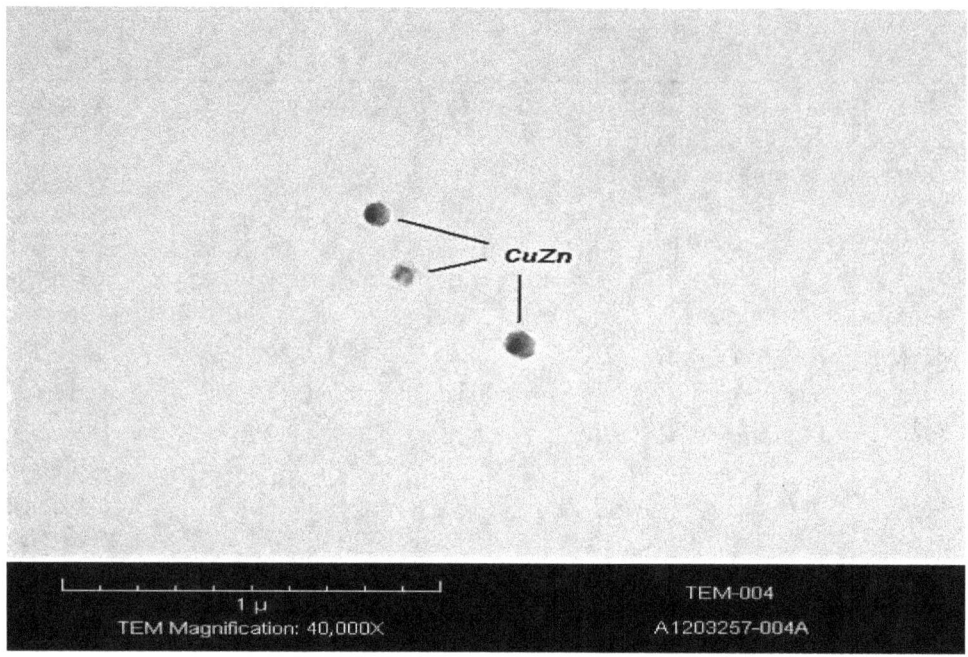

Figure B1. Transmission electron microscope image of particles collected in an instructor's breathing zone during firing of M4 and M9 weapons. Spherical particulate consisting of copper/zinc in the 50–100 nm size range was observed on the MCE filter.

Figure B2. Area particle number concentration within the size range of 20 nm to 1000 nm during the firing of an M4 using the P-Trak instrument.

Figure B3. Area particle mass concentration (mg/m^3) during firing of an M4 using the Dust-Trak instrument.

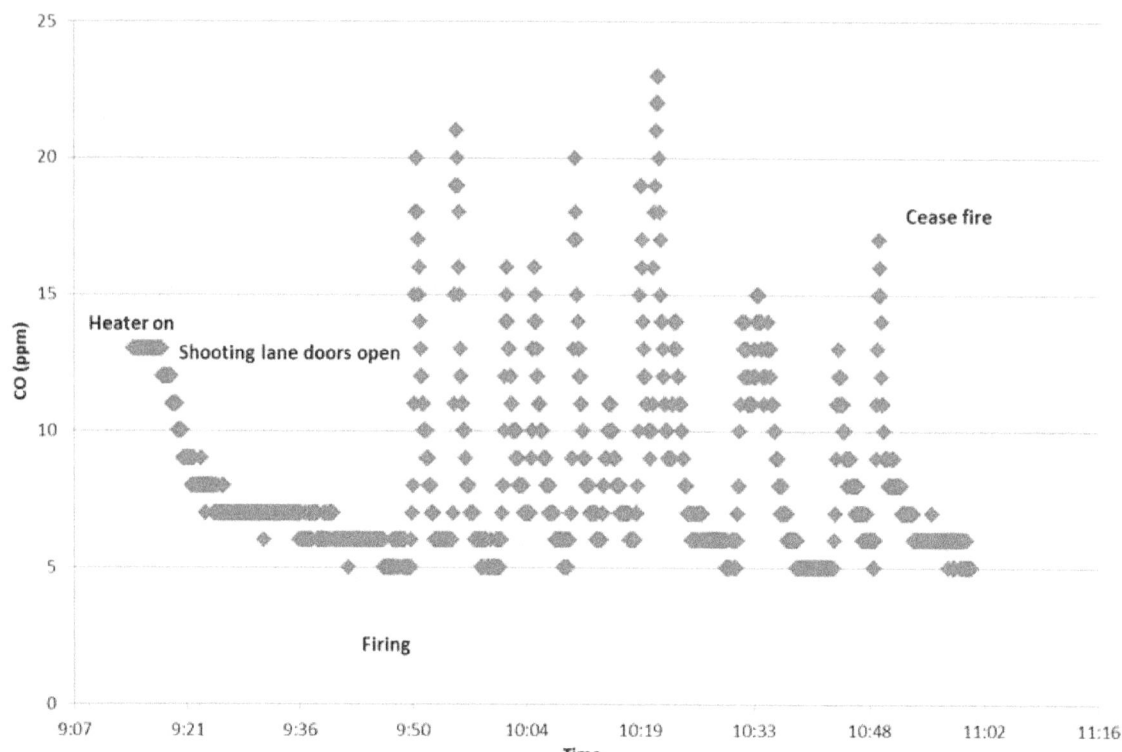

Figure B4. Carbon monoxide concentration inside the range before, during, and after firing events.

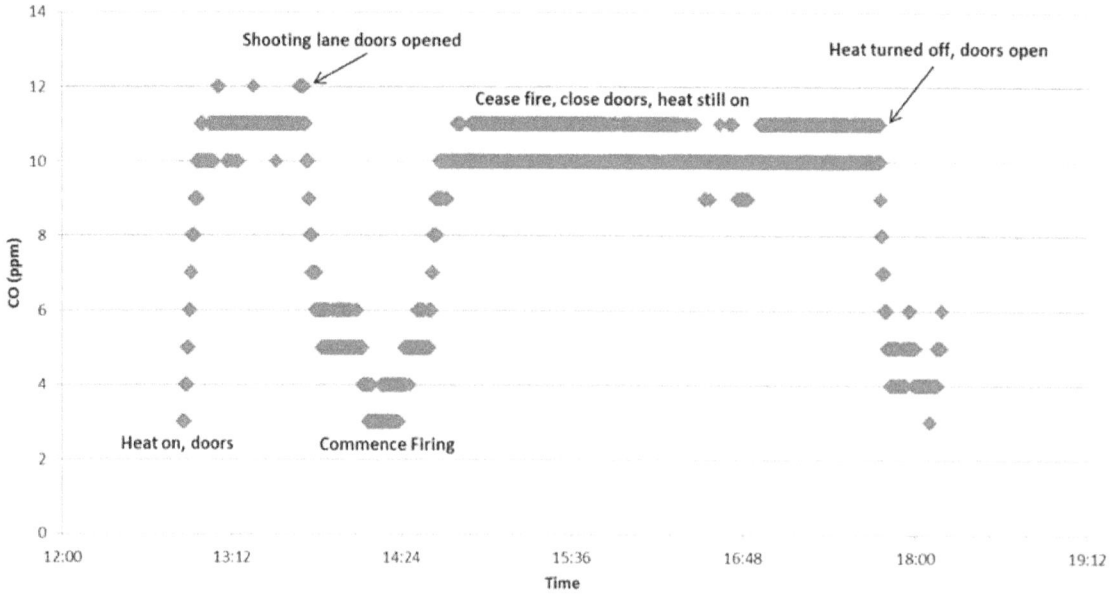

Figure B5. Carbon monoxide concentration inside range before, during and after firing events.

Appendix C: Occupational Exposure Limits and Health Effects

NIOSH investigators refer to mandatory (legally enforceable) and recommended OELs for chemical, physical, and biological agents when evaluating workplace hazards. OELs have been developed by federal agencies and safety and health organizations to prevent adverse health effects from workplace exposures. Generally, OELs suggest levels of exposure that most employees may be exposed to for up to 10 hours per day, 40 hours per week, for a working lifetime, without experiencing adverse health effects. However, not all employees will be protected if their exposures are maintained below these levels. Some may have adverse health effects because of individual susceptibility, a pre-existing medical condition, or a hypersensitivity (allergy). In addition, some hazardous substances act in combination with other exposures, with the general environment, or with medications or personal habits of the employee to produce adverse health effects. Most OELs address airborne exposures, but some substances can be absorbed directly through the skin and mucous membranes.

Most OELs are expressed as a TWA exposure. A TWA refers to the average exposure during a normal 8- to 10-hour workday. Some chemical substances and physical agents have recommended short-term exposure limit or ceiling values. Unless otherwise noted, the short-term exposure limit is a 15-minute TWA exposure. It should not be exceeded at any time during a workday. The ceiling limit should not be exceeded at any time.

In the United States, OELs have been established by federal agencies, professional organizations, state and local governments, and other entities. Some OELs are legally enforceable limits; others are recommendations.

- The U.S. Department of Labor OSHA PELs (29 CFR 1910 [general industry]; 29 CFR 1926 [construction industry]; and 29 CFR 1917 [maritime industry]) are legal limits. These limits are enforceable in workplaces covered under the Occupational Safety and Health Act of 1970.

- NIOSH RELs are recommendations based on a critical review of the scientific and technical information and the adequacy of methods to identify and control the hazard. NIOSH RELs are published in the *NIOSH Pocket Guide to Chemical Hazards* [NIOSH 2010]. NIOSH also recommends risk management practices (e.g., engineering controls, safe work practices, employee education/training, personal protective equipment, and exposure and medical monitoring) to minimize the risk of exposure and adverse health effects.

- Other OELs commonly used and cited in the United States include the TLVs, which are recommended by ACGIH, a professional organization, and the WEELs, which are recommended by the American Industrial Hygiene Association, another professional organization. The TLVs and WEELs are developed by committee members of these associations from a review of the published, peer-reviewed literature. These OELs are not consensus standards. TLVs are considered voluntary exposure guidelines for use by industrial hygienists and others trained in this discipline "to assist in the control of health hazards" [ACGIH 2013]. WEELs have been established for some chemicals "when no other legal or authoritative limits exist" [AIHA 2011].

Outside the United States, OELs have been established by various agencies and organizations and include legal and recommended limits. The Institut für Arbeitsschutz der Deutschen Gesetzlichen Unfallversicherung (Institute for Occupational Safety and Health of the German Social Accident Insurance) maintains a database of international OELs from European Union member states, Canada (Québec), Japan, Switzerland, and the United States. The database, available at http://www.dguv.de/ifa/en/gestis/limit_values/index.jsp, contains international limits for more than 1,500 hazardous substances and is updated periodically.

OSHA requires an employer to furnish employees a place of employment free from recognized hazards that cause or are likely to cause death or serious physical harm [Occupational Safety and Health Act of 1970 (Public Law 91–596, sec. 5(a)(1))]. This is true in the absence of a specific OEL. It also is important to keep in mind that OELs may not reflect current health-based information.

When multiple OELs exist for a substance or agent, NIOSH investigators generally encourage employers to use the lowest OEL when making risk assessment and risk management decisions. NIOSH investigators also encourage use of the hierarchy of controls approach to eliminate or minimize workplace hazards. This includes, in order of preference, the use of (1) substitution or elimination of the hazardous agent, (2) engineering controls (e.g., local exhaust ventilation, process enclosure, dilution ventilation), (3) administrative controls (e.g., limiting time of exposure, employee training, work practice changes, medical surveillance), and (4) personal protective equipment (e.g., respiratory protection, gloves, eye protection, hearing protection). Control banding, a qualitative risk assessment and risk management tool, is a complementary approach to protecting employee health. Control banding focuses on how broad categories of risk should be managed. Information on control banding is available at http://www.cdc.gov/niosh/topics/ctrlbanding/. This approach can be applied in situations where OELs have not been established or can be used to supplement existing OELs.

Below we provide the OELs and surface contamination limits for some of the compounds we measured, as well as a discussion of the potential health effects from exposure to these compounds.

Copper Particulate (as fume or dust/mist)

Copper is a widely used metal that is capable of forming numerous alloys. One of the potential uses of the metal is to form an alloy using zinc which can then be used to produce frangible ammunition. Based on the measurements from this evaluation, under weapon firing conditions of high heat, pressure, and mechanical abrasion, copper-based frangible ammunition can produce fume and nano-sized and larger particulate. The OSHA PEL and the NIOSH REL for copper fume is 0.1 mg/m^3, and 1 mg/m^3 as a dust or mist [NIOSH 2010]. The ACGIH TLV is 0.2 mg/m^3 for the fume and 1 mg/m^3 for the dust or mist [ACGIH 2013].

Health effects from copper fume consist of upper respiratory irritation, metallic taste, nausea, metal fume fever, and possibly discoloration of the hair and skin [ACGIH 2007]. One study identified a condition similar to metal fume fever in workers exposed to metallic copper dust in concentrations on the order of 0.1 mg/m^3 [Gleason 1968]. However, extensive industrial experience related to copper welding and refining in Great Britain indicated that no ill effects result from exposures to fumes at concentrations up to 0.4 mg/m^3 [Luxon 1972].

Carbon Monoxide

CO is a colorless, odorless, tasteless gas produced by incomplete burning of carbon-containing materials such as gasoline or propane fuel. The initial symptoms of CO poisoning may include headache, dizziness, drowsiness, or nausea. Symptoms may advance to vomiting, loss of consciousness, and collapse if prolonged or high exposures are encountered. If the exposure level is high, loss of consciousness may occur without other symptoms. Coma or death may occur if high exposures continue [ACGIH 2007]. The display of symptoms varies widely from individual to individual, and may occur sooner in susceptible individuals such as young or aged people, people with preexisting lung or heart disease, or those living at high altitudes.

The NIOSH REL for CO is 35 ppm for full-shift TWA exposure, with a ceiling limit of 200 ppm that should never be exceeded [NIOSH 1992]. NIOSH has established the immediately dangerous to life or health value for CO as 1,200 ppm [NIOSH 2010]. An immediately dangerous to life or health value is defined as a concentration at which an immediate or delayed threat to life exists or that would interfere with an individual's ability to escape unaided from a space.

The ACGIH recommends an 8-hour TWA TLV of 25 ppm [ACGIH 2013]. ACGIH also recommends that exposures never exceed five times the TLV (thus, never to exceed 125 ppm) [ACGIH 2013]. The OSHA PEL for CO is 50 ppm for an 8-hour TWA exposure [29 CFR 1910.1000].

References

ACGIH [2007]. Documentation of threshold limit values and biological exposure indices. 7th ed. Cincinnati, OH: American Conference of Governmental Industrial Hygienists.

ACGIH [2013]. 2013 TLVs® and BEIs®: threshold limit values for chemical substances and physical agents and biological exposure indices. Cincinnati, OH: American Conference of Governmental Industrial Hygienists.

AFIOH [2008]. Lead free frangible ammunition exposure at United States Air Force small arms firing ranges, 2005–2007. Air Force Institute for Operational Health, Risk Analysis Directorate: United State Air Force. IOH-RS-BR-TR-2008-0002. [http://www.dtic.mil/cgi-bin/GetTRDoc?AD=ADA487506]. Date accessed: July 2013.

AIHA [2011]. AIHA 2011 Emergency response planning guidelines (ERPG) & workplace environmental exposure levels (WEEL) handbook. Fairfax, VA: American Industrial Hygiene Association.

CFR. Code of Federal Regulations. Washington, DC: U.S. Government Printing Office, Office of the Federal Register.

Gleason RP [1968]. Exposure to copper dust. Am Ind Hyg Assoc J *29*(5):461–462.

Luxon SG [1972]. Letter to ACGIH from Industrial Hygiene Unit, H.M. Factory Inspectorate, London, England (August 1, 1972).

Mohlmann C, Aitken RJ, Kenny LC, Gorner P, Vuduc T, Zambelli G [2002]. Size-selective personal air sampling: a new approach using porous foams. Ann Occup Hyg *46*(1):386–389.

NIOSH [1992]. Recommendations for occupational safety and health: compendium of policy documents and statements. By Dames BL. Cincinnati, OH: U.S. Department of Health and Human Services, Centers for Disease Control and Prevention, National Institute for Occupational Safety and Health, DHHS (NIOSH) Publication No. 92-100.

NIOSH [2009]. NIOSH alert: preventing occupational exposures to lead and noise at indoor firing ranges. Cincinnati, OH: U.S. Department of Health and Human Services, Centers for Disease Control and Prevention, National Institute for Occupational Safety and Health, DHHS (NIOSH) Publication No. 2009-136.

NIOSH [2010]. NIOSH pocket guide to chemical hazards. Cincinnati, OH: U.S. Department of Health and Human Services, Centers for Disease Control and Prevention, National Institute for Occupational Safety and Health, DHHS (NIOSH) Publication No. 2010-168c. [http://www.cdc.gov/niosh/npg/]. Date accessed: July 2013.

NIOSH [2013]. NIOSH manual of analytical methods (NMAM®). 4th ed. Schlecht PC, O'Connor PF, eds. Cincinnati, OH: U.S. Department of Health and Human Services, Centers for Disease Control and Prevention, National Institute for Occupational Safety and Health, DHHS (NIOSH) Publication 94-113 (August 1994); 1st Supplement Publication 96-135, 2nd Supplement Publication 98-119; 3rd Supplement 2003-154. [http://www.cdc.gov/niosh/docs/2003-154/].

Pettibone J, Adamcakova-Dodd A, Thorne P, O'Shaugnessy P, Weydert J, Grassian V [2008]. Inflammatory response of mice following inhalation exposure to iron and copper nanoparticles. Nanotoxicology 2(4):189–204.

SKC Inc. [2013]. IOM sampler. [http://www.skcinc.com/instructions/1050.pdf]. Date accessed: July 2013.

USN [2002]. Indoor firing ranges industrial hygiene technical guide. U.S. Navy Environmental Health Center. Technical manual NEHC-TM6290.99-10. Portsmouth, VA: U.S. Department of Defense, Department of the Navy. [http://www.med.navy.mil/sites/nmcphc/Documents/policy-and-instruction/ih-indoor-firing-ranges-technical-guide.pdf]. Date accessed: July 2013.

Wang Z, Li N, Zhao J, White J, Qu P, Xing B [2012]. CuO nanoparticle interaction with human epithelial cells: cellular uptake, location, export, and genotoxicity. Chem Res in Toxicol 25(7):1512–1521.

Keywords: North American Industry Classification System 928110 (National Security), copper, frangible ammunition, nanoparticles, weapons emissions, ventilation, carbon monoxide

Acknowledgments

Analytical Support: Bureau Veritas North America
Desktop Publisher: Mary Winfree
Editor: Ellen Galloway
Health Communicator: Stefanie Brown
Logistics: Donnie Booher and Karl Feldmann

Availability of Report

Recommended citation for this report:
NIOSH [2013]. Health hazard evaluation report: evaluation of instructor and range officer exposure to emissions from copper-based frangible ammunition at a military firing range. By Methner M, Gibbins J, Niemeier T. Cincinnati, OH: U.S. Department of Health and Human Services, Centers for Disease Control and Prevention, National Institute for Occupational Safety and Health, NIOSH HETA Report No. 2012-0091-3187.